Addressing Diseases of Poverty

An Initiative to Reduce the Unacceptable Burden of
Neglected Tropical Diseases in the Asia Pacific Region

"The beginning of wisdom is to call things by their right names." - Chinese Proverb

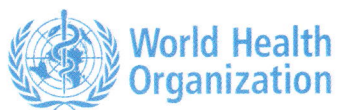
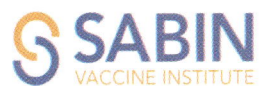
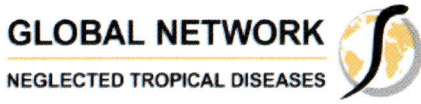
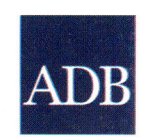

WHO Library Cataloguing-in-Publication Data

Addressing diseases of poverty: an initiative to reduce the unacceptable burden of neglected tropical diseases in the Asia Pacific region.

1. Neglected diseases. 2. Tropical medicine. I. World Health Organization Regional Office for the Western Pacific. II. Asian Development Bank.

ISBN 978 92 9061 651 1 (NLM Classification: WC 680)

© World Health Organization and Asian Development Bank 2014

All rights reserved.

The designations employed and the presentation of the material in this publication do not imply the expression of any opinion whatsoever on the part of the Asian Development Bank and the World Health Organization concerning the legal status of any country, territory, city or area or of its authorities, or concerning the delimitation of its frontiers or boundaries. Dotted lines on maps represent approximate border lines for which there may not yet be full agreement.

This publication follows the World Health Organization practice in reference to its Member States. Where there are space constraints, some country names have been abbreviated. In the Asian Development Bank, China is referred to as the People's Republic of China. The phrases such as "Asia Pacific" and "Asia Pacific region" refer to the Asia and Pacific region. Hong Kong (China) is referred to as "Hong Kong, China" and Macao (China) is referred to as "Macao, China".

The mention of specific companies or of certain manufacturers' products does not imply that they are endorsed or recommended by the Asian Development Bank and the World Health Organization in preference to others of a similar nature that are not mentioned. Errors and omissions excepted, the names of proprietary products are distinguished by initial capital letters.

The Asian Development Bank and the World Health Organization do not warrant that the information contained in this publication is complete and correct and shall not be liable for any damages incurred as a result of its use.

This publication can be obtained from Marketing and Dissemination, World Health Organization, 20 Avenue Appia, 1211 Geneva 27, Switzerland (tel: +41 22 791 2476; fax: +41 22 791 4857; e-mail: bookorders@who.int) and from the Department of External Relations, Asian Development Bank. (fax: +63 2 636 2648; e-mail: adbpub@adb.org).

The Asian Development Bank encourages printing or copying information exclusively for personal and noncommercial use with proper acknowledgment of the Asian Development Bank. Users are restricted from reselling, redistributing, or creating derivative works for commercial purposes without the express, written consent of the Asian Development Bank Requests for permission to reproduce World Health Organization publications, in part or in whole, or to translate them – whether for sale or for noncommercial distribution – should be addressed to Publications, at the above address (fax: +41 22 791 4806; e-mail: permissions@who.int). For World Health Organization Western Pacific Regional Publications, request for permission to reproduce should be addressed to Publications Office, World Health Organization, Regional Office for the Western Pacific, P.O. Box 2932, 1000, Manila, Philippines. (fax: +63 2 5211036; e-mail: publications@wpro.who.int).

Contents

Foreword	iv
Acknowledgements	vi
Abbreviations	vii
Executive summary	viii
Background	1
What are NTDs?	1
Why are NTDs neglected?	4
What is the social and economic impact of NTDs?	4
What is the strategy to reduce the burden of NTDs?	6
Asia Pacific NTD Initiative	9
The Asia Pacific region	9
Asia Pacific NTD Initiative strategy	10
End targets of the Asia Pacific NTD Initiative	11
The partners	12
Potential funding mechanisms	14
Financial resource requirements	15
Why invest in a regional NTD initiative?	17
Investing in the region: Building on existing success	18
References	20
Appendix A: NTDs by country	22
Appendix B: Disease profiles	24
Foodborne trematodiases (FBT)	24
Leishmaniasis	25
Leprosy	26
Lymphatic filariasis (LF)	27
Schistosomiasis	28
Soil-transmitted helminthiases (STH)	29
Trachoma	30
Yaws	31
Other NTDs	32
Appendix C: Specific resource requirements	34

Foreword

Many countries in the Asia Pacific region continue to show impressive economic growth and development despite the turmoil facing much of the world, raising the standard of living for millions of people. However, amid this growth, more than a billion people remain left behind because of widening disparities and unequal access to opportunities for health, development and prosperity. These are the people who are most vulnerable to diseases resulting from poverty, including neglected tropical diseases (NTDs).

Common NTDs trap communities in a cycle of malnutrition and anaemia, poor learning, lower productivity and poor maternal and child health outcomes and, depending on the type of NTD, complications and disabilities such as blindness, swelling of limbs, organ failure or brain damage.

NTD elimination and control efforts are recognized as one of the most cost-effective interventions in global health today. In addition to preventing and reducing disease and disability, NTD elimination and control efforts help maximize the impact of cross-sectoral programmes. These programmes include education, water and sanitation, food safety, nutrition and climate change adaptation. It is critical to work across sectors and leverage integrated approaches at a time when donors, policy-makers and programme managers must improve efficiency to achieve scale and impact with limited resources.

This publication underscores the importance of tackling NTDs in order to help alleviate suffering, reduce poverty and ensure the continued social and economic growth of the region. As a joint production by the World Health Organization Regional Offices for South-East Asia and the Western Pacific, the Asian Development Bank and the Global Network for Neglected Tropical Diseases at the Sabin Vaccine Institute, this publication highlights the need for greater cross-sectoral partnership and additional investments.

The Asia Pacific region has achieved remarkable success in tackling these debilitating diseases under the leadership of governments in endemic countries and with the support of partners worldwide. Lymphatic filariasis has been eliminated in three countries and 10 others are awaiting verification of elimination or are in the surveillance stage before verification by 2016. WHO targets for deworming school-age children have been reached in five countries, and trachoma elimination is expected to be achieved in six countries by 2016.

But these successes are not a reason for complacency. Instead, now is the time to ensure that the investments of the last decade are not wasted. We need to finish the job for some NTDs, such as eliminating lymphatic filariasis and leprosy, and must push for much greater efforts on the ground for others such as schistosomiasis, trachoma, yaws and soil-transmitted helminthiasis. We call on national public and private sectors, bilateral and international agencies and academic institutions and nongovernmental organizations to renew their commitments and expand their investments at this critical juncture.

The fight against NTDs is the first and most fundamental step in ensuring that the most marginalized people will be able to contribute to and participate in the growth and success of countries in the Asia Pacific region. We hope you will join us in despatching NTDs to where they belong—in the history books.

Shin Young-soo, MD, Ph.D.
Regional Director for the Western Pacific
World Health Organization

Samlee Plianbangchang, MD, Dr.PH.
Regional Director for South-East Asia
World Health Organization

Ambassador Michael W. Marine
Chief Executive Officer
Global Network for Neglected Tropical Diseases, Sabin Vaccine Institute

WooChong Um
Officer-in-Charge
Regional and Sustainable Development Department, Asian Development Bank

Acknowledgements

This publication is the outcome of a technical consultation involving the Asian Development Bank, the Global Network for Neglected Tropical Diseases at the Sabin Vaccine Institute and the WHO Regional Office for the Western Pacific. It presents an overview of the burden of neglected tropical diseases in the Asia Pacific region and suggests a way forward.

The publication was developed by the Malaria and other Vectorborne and Parasitic diseases unit of the WHO Regional Office for the Western Pacific and is based on WHO's Regional Strategic Plan for Integrated Neglected Tropical Diseases Control in the South-East Asia Region, 2012–2016 and the Regional Action Plan for Neglected Tropical Diseases in the Western Pacific (2012–2016).

We acknowledge with thanks the contributions of Molly Brady, who drafted the document, and the many people who participated in the collection and analysis of information in this publication and provided valuable feedback, including Padmasiri Eswara Aratchige, Maria Gemma Cabanos, Eva Maria Christophel, Aditya Prasad Dash, Niño Dal Dayanghirang, Marcia de Souza Lima, Vincent de Wit, John Ehrenberg, Bernhard Liese, Amanda Miller, Andreas Mueller, Katsunori Osuga, Kapa Dasaradha Ramaiah, Chandrakant Revankar, Anupama Tantri, Le Anh Tuan, Catharina van Weezenbeek, relevant national programme managers and WHO country offices colleagues in the Western Pacific and South-East Asia regions.

The following individuals reviewed the publication and provided important assistance and feedback: Peter Cordingley, Glenda Gonzales, Silvia Kirchhof, Michael W. Marine, Raymond Mendoza, Neeraj Mistry, Patricia Moser, and Joshua Nealon.

The report was edited by Richard C. Gross. The cover was designed by Rocilyn Laccay and the layout was done by Aileen Magparangalan.

The publication of this report was financed by the Asian Development Bank.

Abbreviations

ADB — Asian Development Bank
FBT — foodborne trematodiases
LF — lymphatic filariasis
NTDs — Neglected Tropical Diseases
STH — soil-transmitted helminthiases
WHO — World Health Organization

Executive summary

The Asia Pacific region is at the forefront of global economic development. Yet some countries and population groups are being left behind in poverty. One of the factors impeding development is a large burden of communicable diseases, especially in vulnerable populations, which perpetuates the cycle of poverty and poor health. Much of this burden can be attributed to neglected tropical diseases (NTDs), a group of diseases caused by many different organisms.

These diseases are present in at least 39 countries and areas in the Asia Pacific, and more than 1 billion people are at risk of infection with at least one. Some NTDs, such as soil-transmitted helminthiases (intestinal worms) and foodborne trematodiases (liver and lung flukes), can be controlled easily at low cost, while others, such as leprosy, lymphatic filariasis (elephantiasis), schistosomiasis (snail fever), trachoma and yaws can even be eliminated.

Left untreated, NTD infections can cause blindness, cognitive impairments, limitations in psychomotor development and disfigurement. Families suffer as those affected members lose their ability to work and take part in social life. Entire communities bear the economic burden from increased health-care costs and reduced productivity. However, proven strategies exist to prevent and treat NTDs. Five of these diseases can be treated properly for less than US$ 0.25 per person through mass distribution of donated medicines to communities at risk; others require diagnosis and treatment delivered through primary health-care services.

The Asia Pacific NTD Initiative was created to support countries in decreasing the burden of NTDs and thereby to reduce suffering and increase productivity. Minimal investments in capacity-building, integrated planning, monitoring and evaluating and technical assistance to overcome logistical bottlenecks can ensure that governments have the resources to implement activities to prevent and treat NTDs.

The objectives of the initiative are manifold. It aims to strengthen political and partner commitment, advocacy and resource mobilization; enhance country capacity in NTD programme management and intersectoral collaboration; scale up access to quality NTD prevention and case management interventions; strengthen integrated NTD surveillance, monitoring and evaluation; and strengthen research capacity and implementation.

With the support of WHO and donors, the Asia Pacific NTD Initiative signifies a call to action for reducing the disproportionate burden of NTDs in the Asia and Pacific region and therefore contributing to poverty reduction in the region. The five-year Asia Pacific NTD Initiative for the control and elimination of NTDs, which highlights successes, priorities and needs, has been costed at US$ 243 million (see Appendix A).

Significant government ownership through budgetary and policy commitments and donor contributions account for nearly 50% of the total budget. The support of pharmaceutical companies and other partners, which donate a substantial proportion of the drugs for these efforts, is key to achieving success. These contributions are appreciated as a shining example of public–private partnerships for development. Yet a gap remains in achieving full access, highlighting yet again the regional health inequities. To ensure the Asia Pacific region reduces the unacceptable burden of NTDs, the support of donors, the private sector and academic and research institutions to close the US$ 121 million gap is crucial.

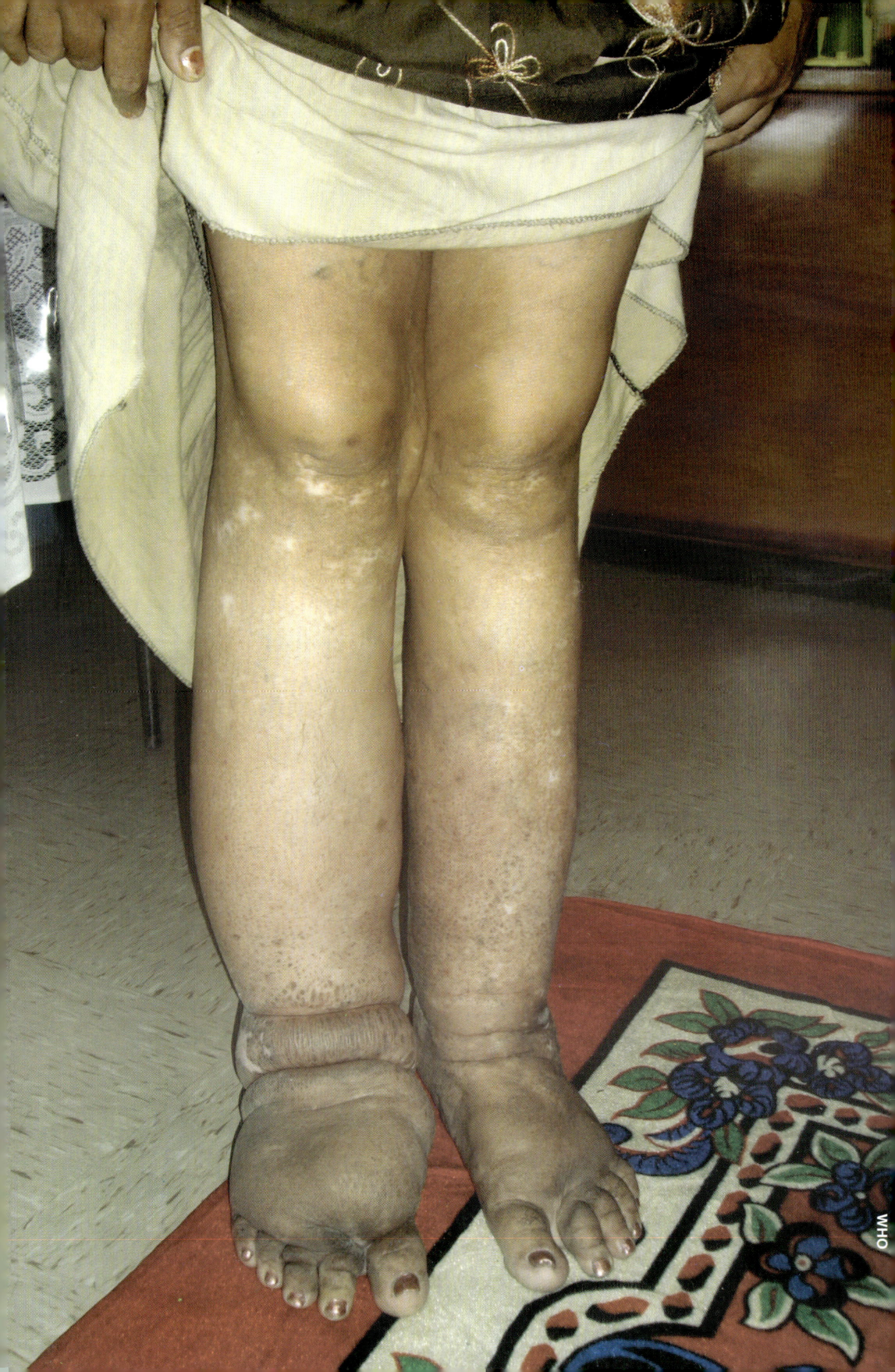

Background

The Asia Pacific region is the area of highest economic growth in the world. Yet some countries and populations are being left behind and still suffer from a high burden of communicable diseases. Many of these diseases, known as neglected tropical diseases (NTDs), have simple and low-cost solutions to reduce their burden.

NTDs are comprised of 17 medically diverse diseases that threaten over 1 billion people in the Asia Pacific region, most of whom live on less than US$ 1.25 a day. NTDs stigmatize and disable, preventing individuals from being able to care for themselves or their families. They impair physical and cognitive development, cause adverse pregnancy outcomes and limit adult productivity in the workforce. As a result, they cause billions of dollars in lost wages, all but ensuring those infected and their family members remain trapped in a cycle of poverty and disease.

The Asia Pacific NTD Initiative seeks to reduce needless suffering and disability by scaling up access to treatment for these diseases. Reducing the burden of NTDs is an integral part of improving maternal and child health. With a little external investment, this cycle of disease, which continues to keep so many people in poverty, can be broken.

What are NTDs?

NTDs are diseases caused by parasites, bacteria, viruses and other organisms. The most common NTDs in the Asia Pacific region are lymphatic filariasis (LF), trachoma, yaws, leprosy, leishmaniasis, soil-transmitted helminthiases (STH), schistosomiasis and foodborne trematodiases (FBT).

Some of these diseases can be eliminated by breaking cycles of transmission, including LF/elephantiasis, trachoma, schistosomiasis/snail fever, yaws, leprosy and leishmaniasis/kala azar. Others can be addressed through strategies to reduce the burden of disease but need longer-term support from multiple sectors to achieve sustainable disease control. These include STH/intestinal worms and FBT/liver and lung flukes.

Opposite page: A female patient with elephantiasis in Fiji.

Moving towards elimination

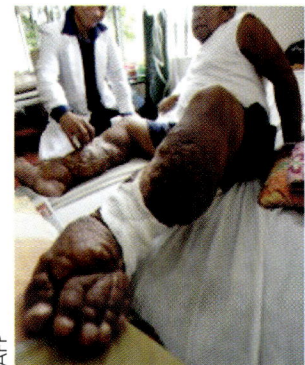

LF/elephantiasis: Three countries in the Asia Pacific region – China, the Republic of Korea and Solomon Islands – have been verified as having eliminated LF as a public health problem, a disabling disease caused by filarial worms transmitted by mosquitoes. Eleven more countries are in the process of verifying elimination, 17 are distributing medicines to endemic communities and three are assessing endemicity status. In addition, people suffering from chronic diseases related to LF, such as lymphoedema and scrotal swelling, still need access to chronic care and surgery.

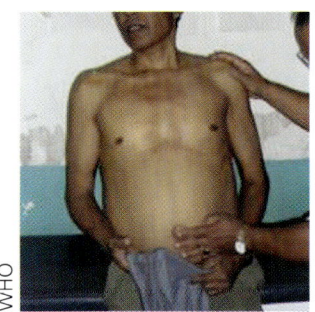

Schistosomiasis/snail fever: Schistosomiasis, caused by a worm found in contaminated fresh water, occurs in five countries in the region. Varying types of schistosomiasis can cause symptoms that include abdominal pain, diarrhoea, malnutrition and severe liver pathology.

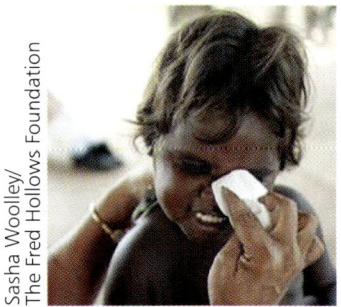

Trachoma: Tools exist to effectively treat and prevent the spread of trachoma, a bacterial infection that is a leading cause of preventable blindness. However, the disease remains endemic in at least 14 countries and areas in the region.

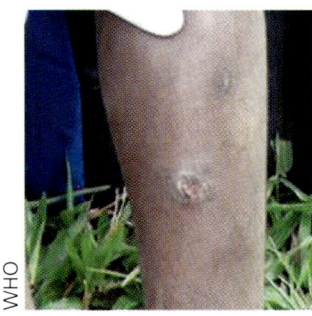

Yaws: Yaws occurs among poor populations in remote areas in Indonesia, Papua New Guinea, Solomon Islands, Timor-Leste and Vanuatu. It is a chronic bacterial infection that affects mainly the skin, bone and cartilage; however, it can be treated with a single injection of penicillin. A new strategy to eliminate the disease, an oral administration of azithromycin, is being piloted in highly endemic communities.

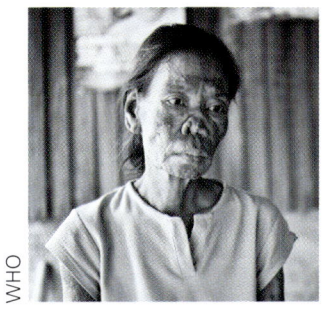
Leprosy: Leprosy, a bacterial disease that causes disability and disfigurement, has been eliminated as public health problem (less than one case per 10 000 population) at a regional level in the Asia Pacific. Although "elimination status" has been maintained, large numbers of new cases are still reported in countries like China, India and the Philippines, which need support for early case detection and multidrug therapy.

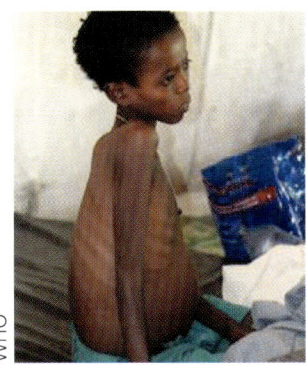
Leishmaniasis/kala azar: Leishmaniasis is endemic in five countries in the region. It is caused by parasites transmitted through the bites of sand flies and is usually fatal if left untreated. Transmission can be reduced through active case detection and early treatment as well as vector control.

Working towards sustainable control

STH/intestinal worms: Infection with intestinal worms is an underlying cause of poor physical and cognitive development in children and anaemia in pregnant women. Over 471 million children require deworming in at least 25 countries and areas in the region (see Appendix A). Countries like Cambodia – the first country in the world to reach the WHO target of treatment of 75% of school-age children at risk for STH – have shown that, with a small amount of resources, it is possible to achieve this goal.

FBT/liver and lung flukes: To control foodborne trematode infections, caused by eating food infected with worms, habits such as eating raw fish need to be changed in the nine endemic countries in the region. The priority is to treat infected people now while working toward longer-term solutions of changing eating habits, improving sanitation and strengthening food safety.

Why are NTDs neglected?

Given the debilitating effects of NTDs, it is important to understand why NTDs do not receive adequate attention or funding. NTDs are, indeed, neglected for the following reasons:

- These diseases predominantly affect people who are living in areas of poverty or in population groups in remote, hard-to-reach, inaccessible areas and whose problems are rarely highlighted.
- Control efforts for NTDs compete with other public health priorities such as HIV, tuberculosis, malaria and emerging infectious diseases for funding from the international community. Unlike those diseases, NTDs do not generally threaten the population of donor countries.
- The social and economic burden of NTDs is hidden as they generally cause low mortality and do not usually result in outbreaks. They do, however, insidiously rob people of their capacity to be productive members of society.
- There is not enough awareness of the possibilities of integrating NTD control and elimination activities into cross-sectoral interventions.

What is the social and economic impact of NTDs?

NTDs are a serious obstacle to economic development in many low-income nations. Although NTDs do not often affect people living in high-income countries, they result in billions of dollars of lost wages and economic productivity and trap endemic communities in a cycle of poverty and disease (Conteh, Engels & Molyneux, 2010). In infected individuals, they cause physical and cognitive development impairments and often result in discrimination against those who develop disfigurement (Addiss & Brady, 2007; Bethony et al., 2006; Weiss, 2008).

NTDs, such as STH, schistosomiasis and LF, often occur in remote areas and impoverished environments. If social and economic development leads to significant improvements in living conditions and hygiene, these diseases will gradually disappear.

Box 1 Social and economic impact of NTDs

- Soil-transmitted helminth infections disproportionately affect school-age children, compromising cognitive and physical development, leading to decreased earnings in adulthood (Baird, Hicks, Kremer & Miguel, 2011).
- Poor health among women, from anaemia and malnutrition due to STH infection, as well as clinical disabilities, affects the health and development of entire families (Larocque, Casapia, Gotuzzo, & Gyorkos, 2005).
- In India, chronic LF patients are estimated to lose as much as 11 years of productivity, at US$ 50 lost per year, or 15% of an individual's income (Ramaiah, Das, Michael & Guyatt, 2000).
- Globally, trachoma, which if untreated can cause permanent blindness, is estimated to cause a loss of US$ 5.3 billion annually in agricultural productivity (Frick, Hanson & Jacobson, 2003).

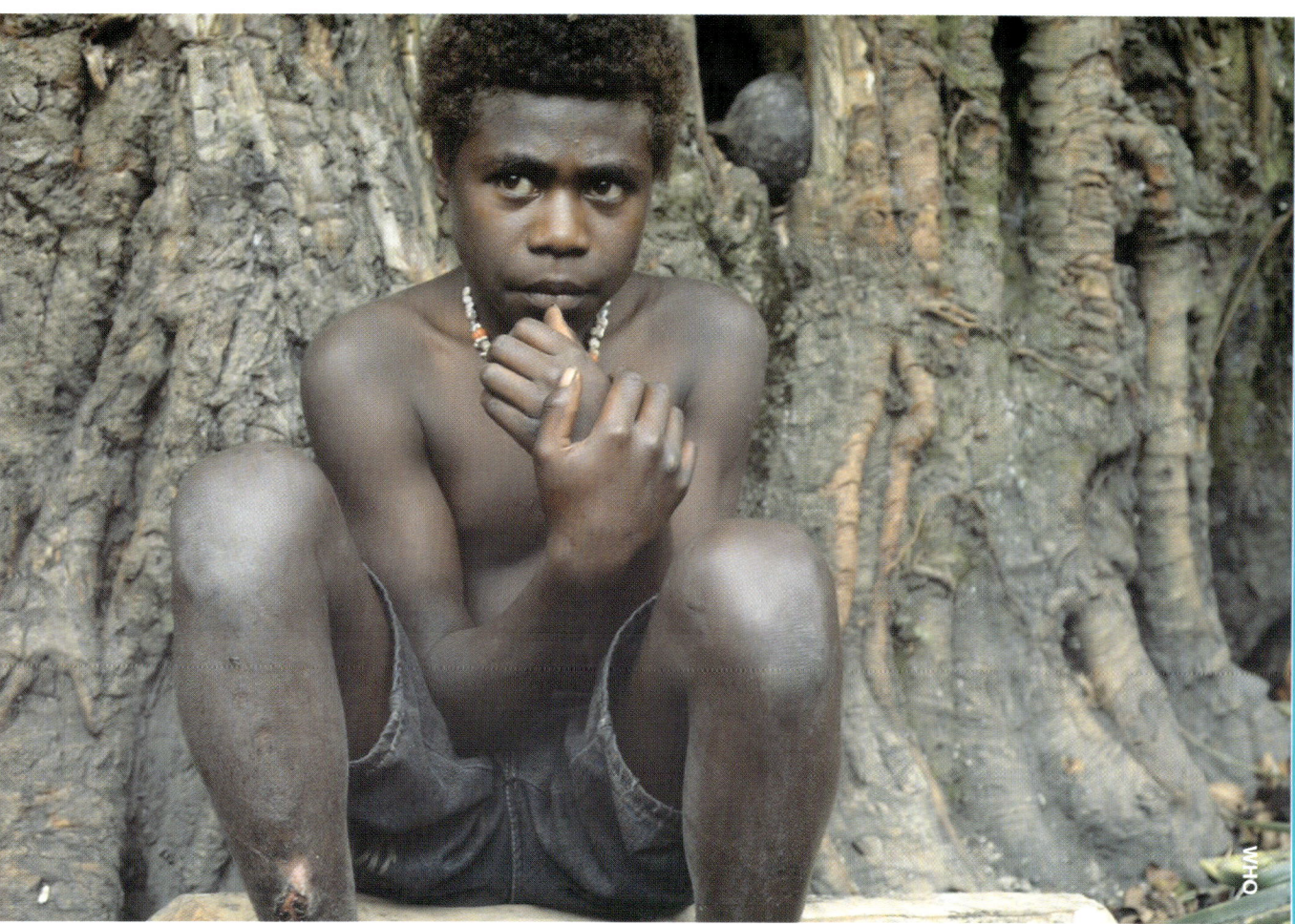

A yaws patient in Vanuatu.

What is the strategy to reduce the burden of NTDs?

The diverse challenges of NTDs call for an overarching strategy to expand access to preventive interventions and strengthen the capacity of primary health care systems to respond to these diseases. Three packages of interventions are needed to control and eliminate the NTDs targeted in this regional programme.

The first, preventive chemotherapy, includes mass distribution of medicines to select populations at regular intervals (World Health Organization, 2006). In the case of LF, trachoma, and yaws, the aim of preventive chemotherapy is to interrupt transmission and eliminate the disease. In the case of STH, schistosomiasis and some FBT, preventive chemotherapy is used to reduce the disease burden. Distribution of medicines can often be combined with other health interventions, such as integrated management of childhood illnesses, immunization campaigns and bednet distribution in malaria-endemic areas.

The second, case management, is used to identify and manage infection and disease in individual patients through the primary health care system. Depending on the disease, activities to support this intervention can include active case finding, active contact tracing, chronic care and treatment and surgery. Case management is the primary intervention for leprosy, some of the FBT, leishmaniasis and other NTDs (see Appendix B).

The third, transmission control, includes cross-cutting intersectoral activities such as health promotion, vector control, water supply and sanitation improvement and food safety improvement. Since some of these diseases occur in both humans and animals, coordination with the veterinary health sector to lower infections in animals is necessary to ensure continued lowered infection rates in people. Improvements in farming practices, such as China's move to replace buffalos (which spread schistosomiasis) with tractors, will help the health sector move towards elimination of this disease. Transmission control interventions are complementary to preventive chemotherapy and case management. For STH, schistosomiasis and FBT, they are essential to sustainable prevention and control as preventive chemotherapy alone will not be enough to interrupt transmission and keep the burden low.

With support from WHO, countries and areas are encouraged to write integrated national NTD plans of action, including activities and costing. This process ensures country ownership of these disease programmes and provides a framework for harmonizing donor contributions. Most importantly, the development of national NTD programmes provides a scaffold for the enhancement of national NTD programme management and implementation capacity, ensures proper monitoring and evaluation of activities and leads to information sharing that increases the efficiency and impact of the funds invested.

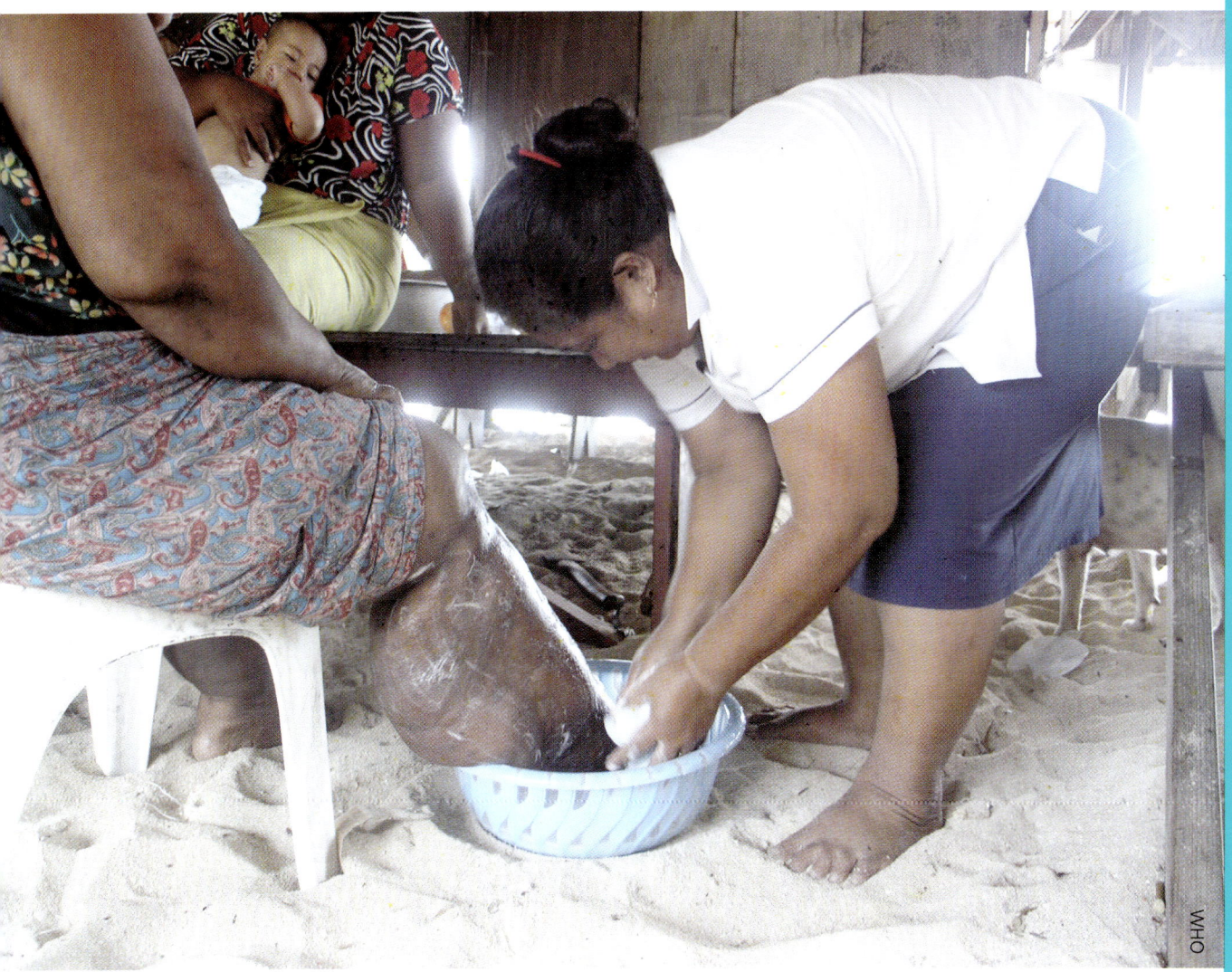

National programme assures individual care to elephantiasis patients in Kiribati.

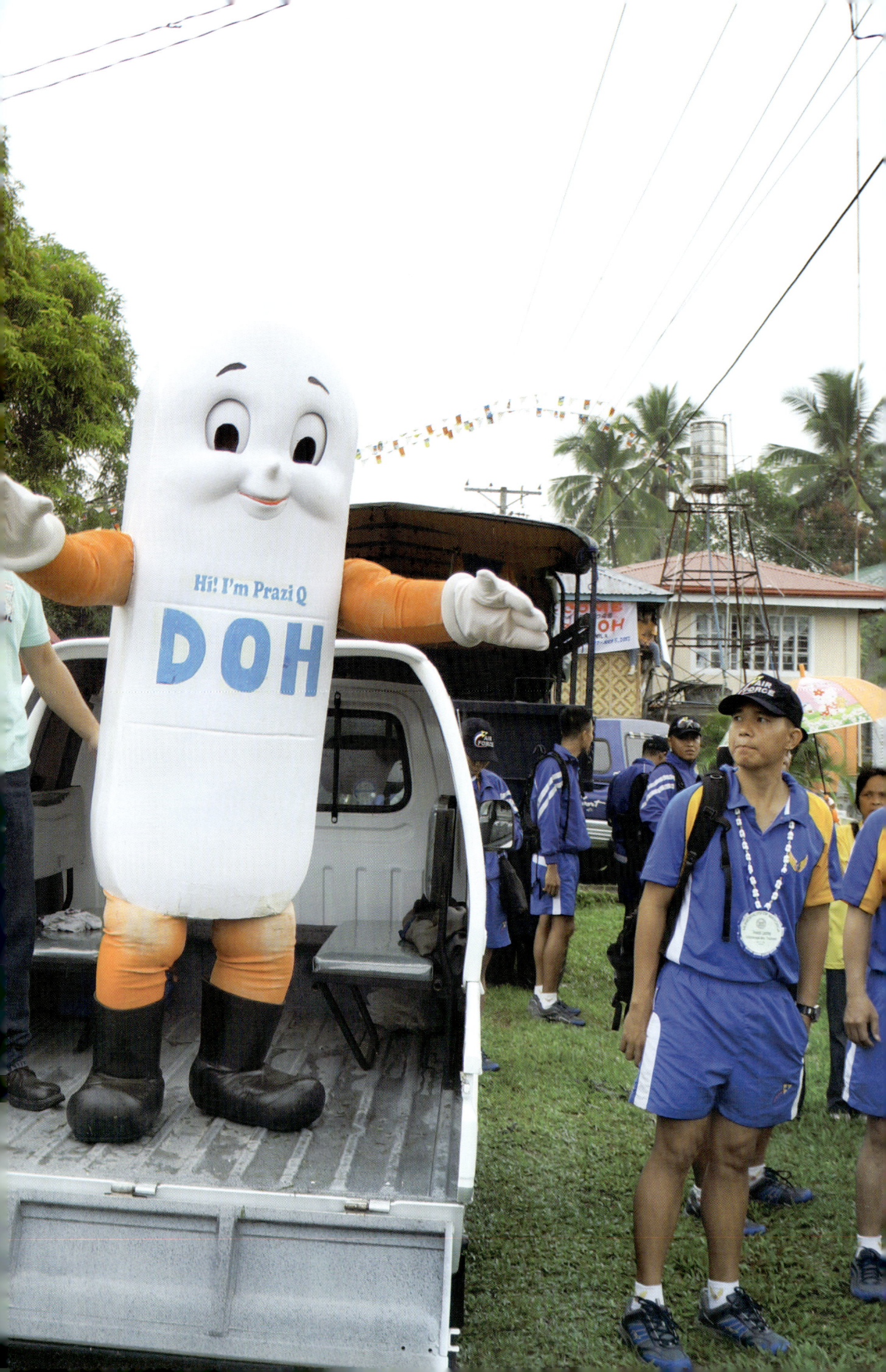

Asia Pacific NTD Initiative

The Asia Pacific NTD Initiative has its foundation in the *WHO Regional Strategic Plan for Integrated NTD Control in the South-East Asia Region (2012–2016)* and the *WHO Regional Action Plan for Neglected Tropical Diseases in the Western Pacific (2012–2016)*. These regional plans are used to formulate national NTD plans of action, monitor programme progress and mobilize internal and external funds.

The Asia Pacific NTD Initiative serves as a framework for countries and areas, donors, research institutes and other partners. It includes support to activities such as:

- programme planning and capacity-building,
- health education,
- mass drug distribution,
- curative care and morbidity management,
- monitoring and evaluation and surveillance, and
- knowledge management and operational research.

The Asia Pacific region

The Asia Pacific NTD Initiative supports countries and areas in WHO's South-East Asia and Western Pacific regions. The Asia Pacific region covers 48 countries and areas and stretches from China in the north, south to New Zealand, west to India, across Indonesia and to French Polynesia in the east. It includes about 3.4 billion people, with populations ranging from China's 1.34 billion people to Pitcairn Islands' 63. The Asia Pacific region is also diverse in terms of income, including high-income countries, rapidly emerging economies and some of the lowest-income countries in the world.

Opposite page: The Department of Health mascot on display during mass treatment for schistosomiasis in the Philippines

Asia Pacific NTD Initiative goals and objectives

The goal of the Asia Pacific NTD Initiative is to reduce the health and socioeconomic impact of NTDs, especially among vulnerable groups, and eliminate specific diseases where feasible. Its objectives are the following:

- **Objective 1:** Strengthen political and partners' commitment, advocacy and resource mobilization for NTDs.

- **Objective 2:** Enhance country capacity for NTD programme management and intersectoral collaboration in order to sustain and scale up NTD programmes.

- **Objective 3:** Scale up access to quality NTD prevention and case management interventions.

- **Objective 4:** Strengthen integrated NTD surveillance, monitoring and evaluation.

- **Objective 5:** Strengthen research capacity on NTDs and implement research to fill programmatic knowledge gaps.

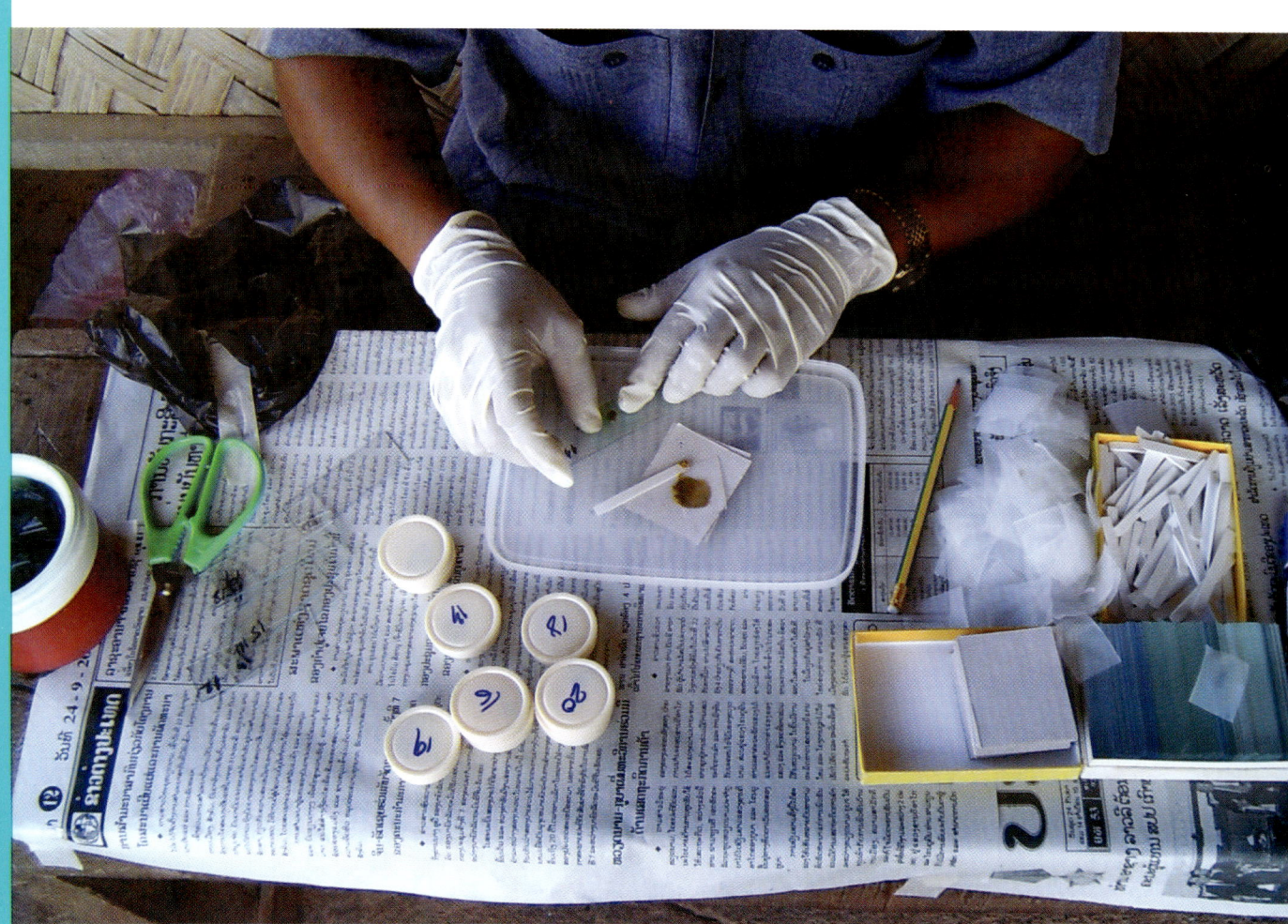

A health worker examining stool for helminthiasis in the Lao People's Democratic Republic.

End targets of the Asia Pacific NTD Initiative

By 2016, the Asia Pacific NTD Initiative aims to accomplish the following:

Eliminating disease

- **LF** will be eliminated[1] in 17 additional countries and areas[2].
- Blinding **trachoma** will be eliminated[3] in six countries: Cambodia, China, the Lao People's Democratic Republic, Myanmar, Nepal and Viet Nam.
- **Schistosomiasis** will be eliminated[4] in four countries: Cambodia, China, Indonesia and the Lao People's Democratic Republic.
- **Yaws** programmes will progress towards elimination[5] in five countries: Indonesia, Papua New Guinea, Solomon Islands, Timor-Leste and Vanuatu.
- **Leprosy** will be eliminated[6] in Kiribati, the Marshall Islands and the Federated States of Micronesia and sustained at below elimination level in all other countries.
- **Leishmaniasis** will be eliminated[7] in five countries: Bangladesh, Bhutan, China, India and Nepal.

Reducing Disease

- Morbidity due to **STH** will be reduced by achieving at least 75% national deworming coverage among school-age children in 20 countries[8] and of preschool-age children in 18 countries[9]. The programme will also build on established systems to expand treatment to women of childbearing age at risk.
- Morbidity due to **FBT** will be reduced through achieving 75% coverage of at-risk population in three countries: the Lao People's Democratic Republic, the Republic of Korea and Viet Nam.

---

[1] LF elimination as a public health problem is defined as the absence of LF transmission, measured in part by <2% antigen prevalence in Culex/Anopheles areas and <1% antigen prevalence in Aedes areas.

[2] American Samoa, Bangladesh, Cambodia, Cook Islands, India, Maldives, the Marshall Islands, Myanmar, Nepal, Niue, Palau, Sri Lanka, Thailand, Tonga, Vanuatu, Viet Nam and Wallis and Futuna

[3] Blinding trachoma elimination is defined as, at a subdistrict level, trachoma follicular prevalence <5% in children aged one to nive years old and, at the district level, less than one trichiasis case unknown to the health system per 1000 population.

[4] Elimination of schistosomiasis as a public health problem is defined as <1% prevalence of heavy-intensity infections in humans in sentinel sites.

[5] Indonesia and Timor-Leste aim to reduce new cases to zero in endemic districts; while Papua New Guinea, Solomon Islands and Vanuatu aim to map the burden of disease and start interventions.

[6] Leprosy elimination as a public health problem is defined as less than one case per 10 000 population.

[7] Leishmaniasis elimination as a public health problem is defined as less than one new case per 10 000 population at risk.

[8] Bangladesh, Bhutan, Cambodia, China, the Democratic People's Republic Korea, Fiji, India, Indonesia, Kiribati, the Lao People's Democratic Republic, Malaysia, the Marshall Islands, Myanmar, Nepal, the Philippines, Timor-Leste, Tonga, Tuvalu, Vanuatu, Viet Nam.

[9] Bangladesh, Bhutan, Cambodia, China, the Democratic People's Republic Korea, Fiji, India, Indonesia, Kiribati, the Lao People's Democratic Republic, Malaysia, Myanmar, Nepal, the Philippines, Timor-Leste, Tonga, Tuvalu, Viet Nam.

The partners

The ministry of health in each country is the lead partner for implementation of national NTD programmes, given its responsibility for mapping, planning and implementing activities. The ministries are encouraged and technically supported by WHO in the process of drafting integrated NTD plans, including budgetary costing for the necessary interventions.

For some NTD activities, the ministry of education plays a crucial part in programme design and implementation. School health initiatives often include deworming and helping countries and areas achieve the World Health Assembly goal of treating 75% of school-age children at risk of infection. Collaboration between ministries of health and education can play a vital role in institutionalizing deworming activities and reducing costs.

However, governments of endemic countries and areas cannot meet their goals alone. Much of the progress in the Asia Pacific against NTDs in the past 10 years has been accomplished as a result of the continued support of valued partners from the private sector (especially pharmaceutical companies making drug donations), bilateral and international agencies, academic institutions and nongovernmental organizations.

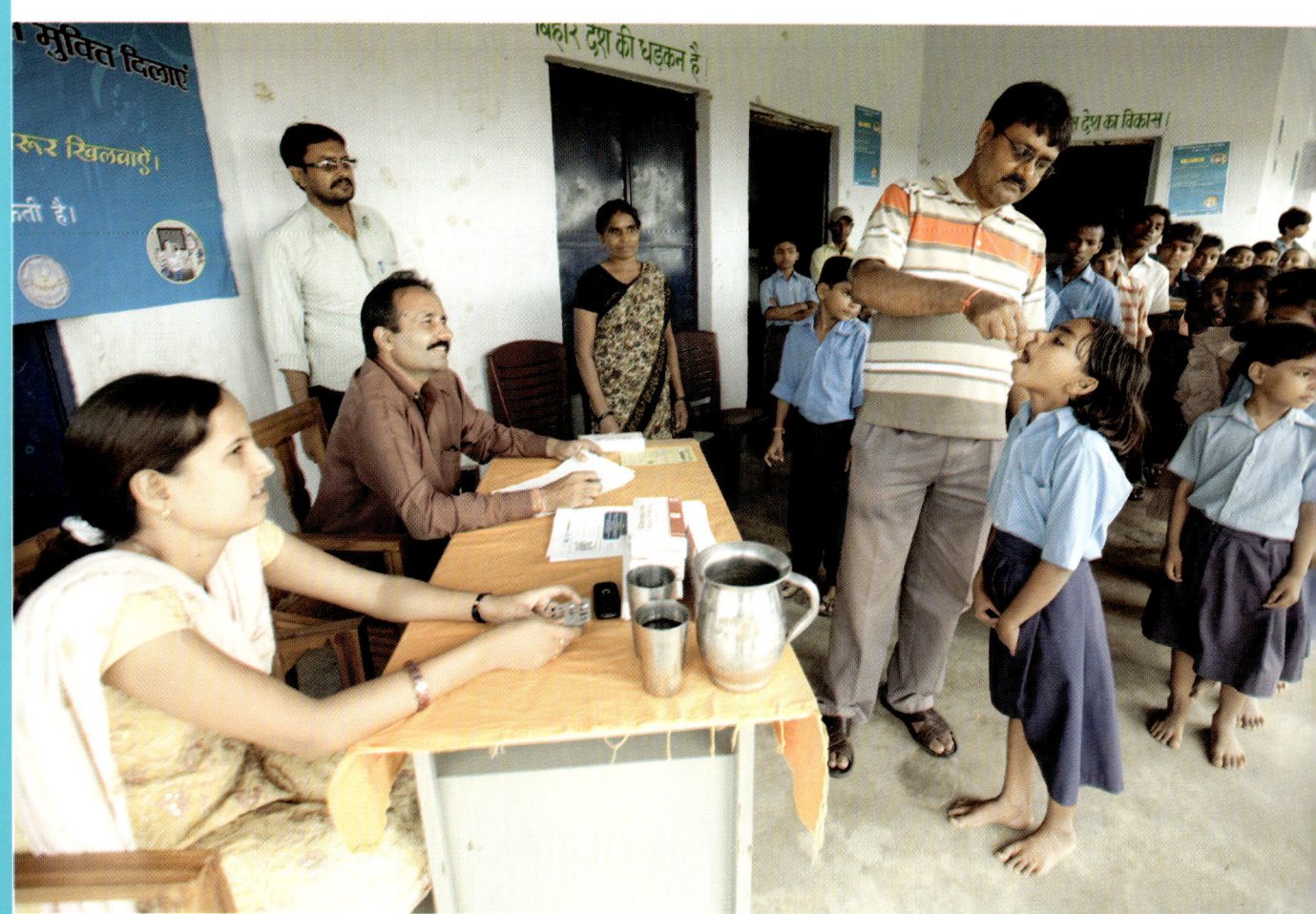

Students from Phulwari Sharif School in Bihar, India participate in a deworming programs.

WHO has provided leadership and technical support for NTD elimination and control efforts. It oversees NTD programme progress through the NTD regional programme review groups, which also approve applications for some of the donated NTD medicines. WHO uses its convening power and close links with ministries of health to bring multiple stakeholders together to plan and implement NTD programmes. Given its expertise in a broad spectrum of health issues, it also helps NTD programmes synergize with other well-established communicable disease interventions.

Bilateral agencies and donor governments in the region have made significant investments and provided tremendous support and technical guidance to endemic countries. As these countries now approach their goals for elimination and control, continued and enhanced commitment from these critical partners is needed.

The Asian Development Bank (ADB) has supported NTD activities in Cambodia, the Lao People's Democratic Republic and Viet Nam as part of a project to strengthen communicable disease surveillance and response systems, improve disease control for vulnerable groups and strengthen regional coordination in disease response.

Civil society and nongovernmental organizations working in the implementation, advocacy and resource mobilization fields are also valued partners.

Potential funding mechanisms

Considerable commitments by endemic countries and areas to NTD programming have been bolstered by the pledges of pharmaceutical companies to donate necessary medicines. Yet there remains a significant funding gap for national programmes to scale up access to prevention and treatment as well as interventions to control transmission. National plans for integrated NTD control can be financed through several modalities, which vary greatly depending on donor involvement, structure and governance.

- **Development bank free-standing NTD projects**
  This mechanism results in projects owned and executed by development banks through a national or regional NTD project. It provides an opportunity for leveraging funds through cofinancing a project with several entities, including development banks and bilateral government contributions. It allows donors to earmark funds for specific programmes, diseases or countries and areas.

- **Add-on NTD components to development projects**
  NTD components can be added on to existing development projects managed by development banks or bilateral agencies. Given the links between health and development, this type of funding can provide a way to use a health lens to monitor and evaluate development and infrastructure programmes in water and sanitation, education, environment and agriculture. Examples of this type of investment could be adding on foodborne trematode disease prevention activities to food safety initiatives, schistosomiasis and trachoma interventions to water and sanitation infrastructure development and deworming programmes to poverty-reduction or education strategies.

- **Direct bilateral support to national NTD programmes**
  Another way to finance NTD activities is to fund governments directly for the purpose of supporting the national NTD programme. Governments of endemic countries and areas have been encouraged to draft national integrated NTD plans of action, which can help to ensure government commitment and sustainability. This provides an opportunity for a very active, involved role for the donors, with more oversight for how funds are allocated and programmes are implemented.

- **Support to national NTD programmes through WHO**
  WHO also supports national programmes by providing technical and financial support. Past funding for NTDs has been channelled through WHO to support planning, implementation and/or NTD programme monitoring. In this case, donors are assured of WHO oversight and technical support for the activities.

- **A multidonor trust fund that pools funding from several sources**
  This funding mechanism allows for the benefit of allocating funds to national governments through a transparent multidonor mechanism. It encourages dialogue with governments, coordinating projects closely and ensuring that NTDs are put on the health agenda leading to a sustainable approach. Proposals would be reviewed by a technical advisory group, including representatives of donors, nongovernmental organizations and WHO. Flexible governance structures allow for donors' participation in annual meetings to assess the design and execution of fund management and to discuss potential problems and solutions. Additionally, donors are able to leverage and share in credit for the cumulative amount of funds deposited into the trust fund as well as all of the activities financed through the fund.

Opposite page: Improving access to clean water in the Lao People's Democratic Republic

Financial resource requirements

The Asia Pacific NTD Initiative is a comprehensive programme that has been planned to support countries and areas over the next five years to move towards the elimination of five NTDs and sustainable control of others. The total budget of this programme is estimated at US$ 243 million, with US$ 122 million already committed by endemic countries and areas, bilateral donors and drug companies.

It has estimated the costs for five years of activities. For countries in the WHO South-East Asia Region, these include budgets and gaps estimated as part of national NTD plans for Bangladesh, Indonesia, Myanmar, Nepal and Timor-Leste as well as the South-East Asia Regional Office. India is not yet included in this budget estimate. The budgets and gaps estimated for the Western Pacific Region exclude budgets for countries and areas which do not need external assistance, such as Brunei Darussalam, China, Japan, the Republic of Korea, Malaysia and New Caledonia.

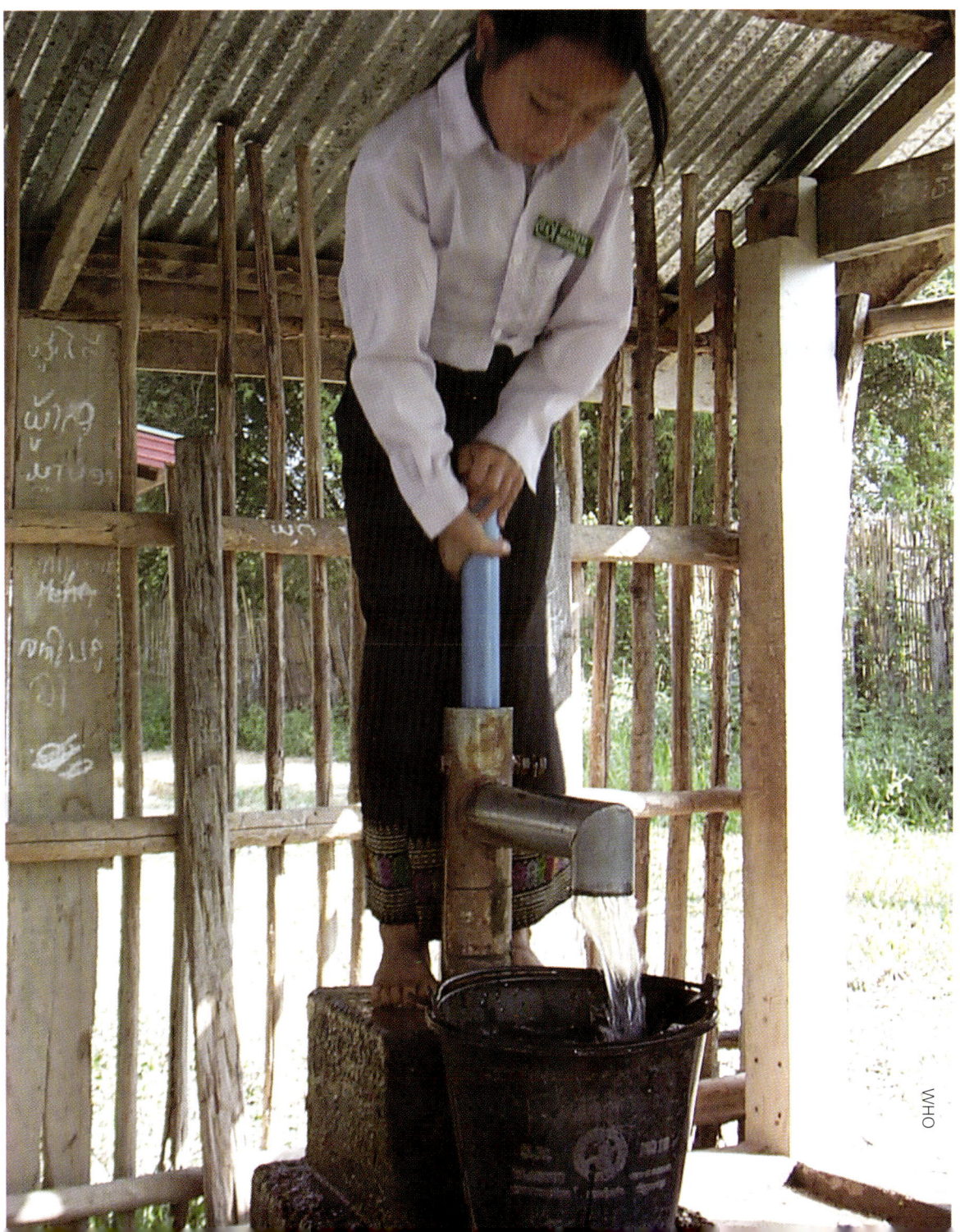

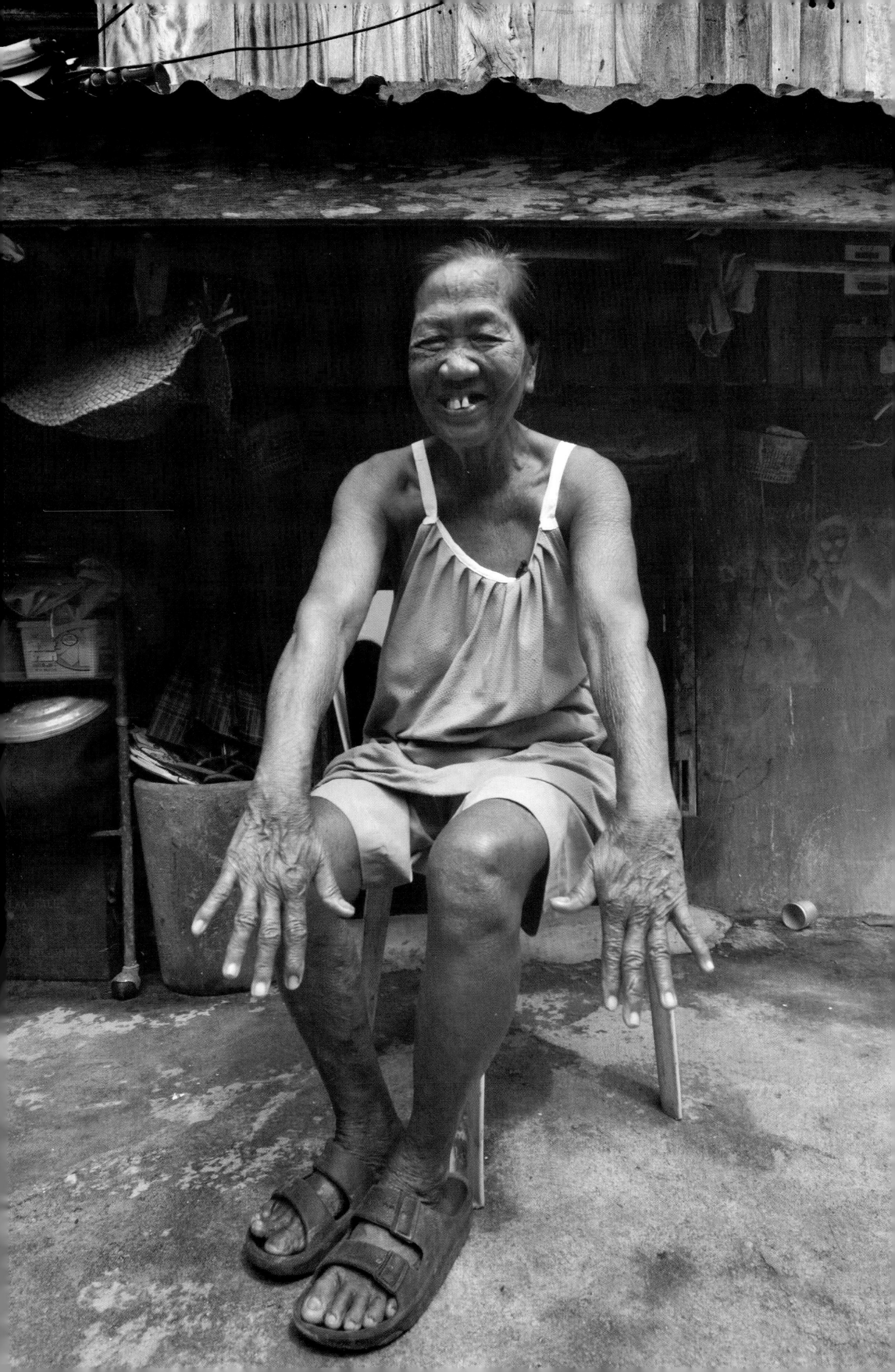

Why invest in a regional NTD initiative?

There are five key reasons why endemic-country governments and donors should invest in a regional NTD programme.

1. Controlling and eliminating NTDs will reduce poverty.

The Asia Pacific NTD Initiative will contribute to poverty reduction in noteworthy ways. Research indicates that NTD control significantly improves maternal health, reduces neonatal mortality, improves childhood growth and development and mitigates chronic, often irreversible, disease at later stages in life (Brooker, Hotez, & Bundy, 2008; Miguel & Kremer, 2004; Ottesen, Hooper, Bradley & Biswas, 2008). Reducing morbidity and new infections leading to disability cuts costs for health care. For example, in the Asia Pacific region, from 2000 to 2007, the LF programme averted US$ 2.12 billion in lifetime health system costs by preventing people from contracting a disabling disease (Chu, Hooper, Bradley, McFarland & Ottesen, 2010). The benefits of NTD control and elimination extend beyond health; increased worker productivity can contribute to growing economies, directly and sustainably contributing to the livelihoods of millions of families. With limited investments, the regional programme will contribute to improving the health status of the over 900 million people at risk in the region, thus also improving their economic situation.

2. NTDs require and promote intersectoral approaches.

Those NTDs, such as STH and foodborne trematodes, which need sustainable control strategies, create opportunities to work intersectorally to improve safe water, sanitation and food safety. NTD activities can be added to other development projects to enhance the impact of poverty-reduction investments by reducing disease such as schistosomiasis control by including better irrigation and mass drug distribution in infrastructure projects.

3. There are evidence-based, low-cost strategies that protect and treat people at risk of NTDs.

NTDs such as STH, LF and schistosomiasis can be prevented with simple and cost-effective interventions. A small amount of external funding can catalyse significant endemic country commitments. Because of the donations of necessary medicines by drug companies, the mass distribution of medicines to communities at risk in the Asia Pacific region costs from US$ 0.02 to US$ 0.19 per person treated when treated in disease-specific campaigns (Goldman et al., 2007; Montresor et al., 2008).

Opposite page: Person affected by leprosy in the Philippines saying, "I am cured of leprosy!"

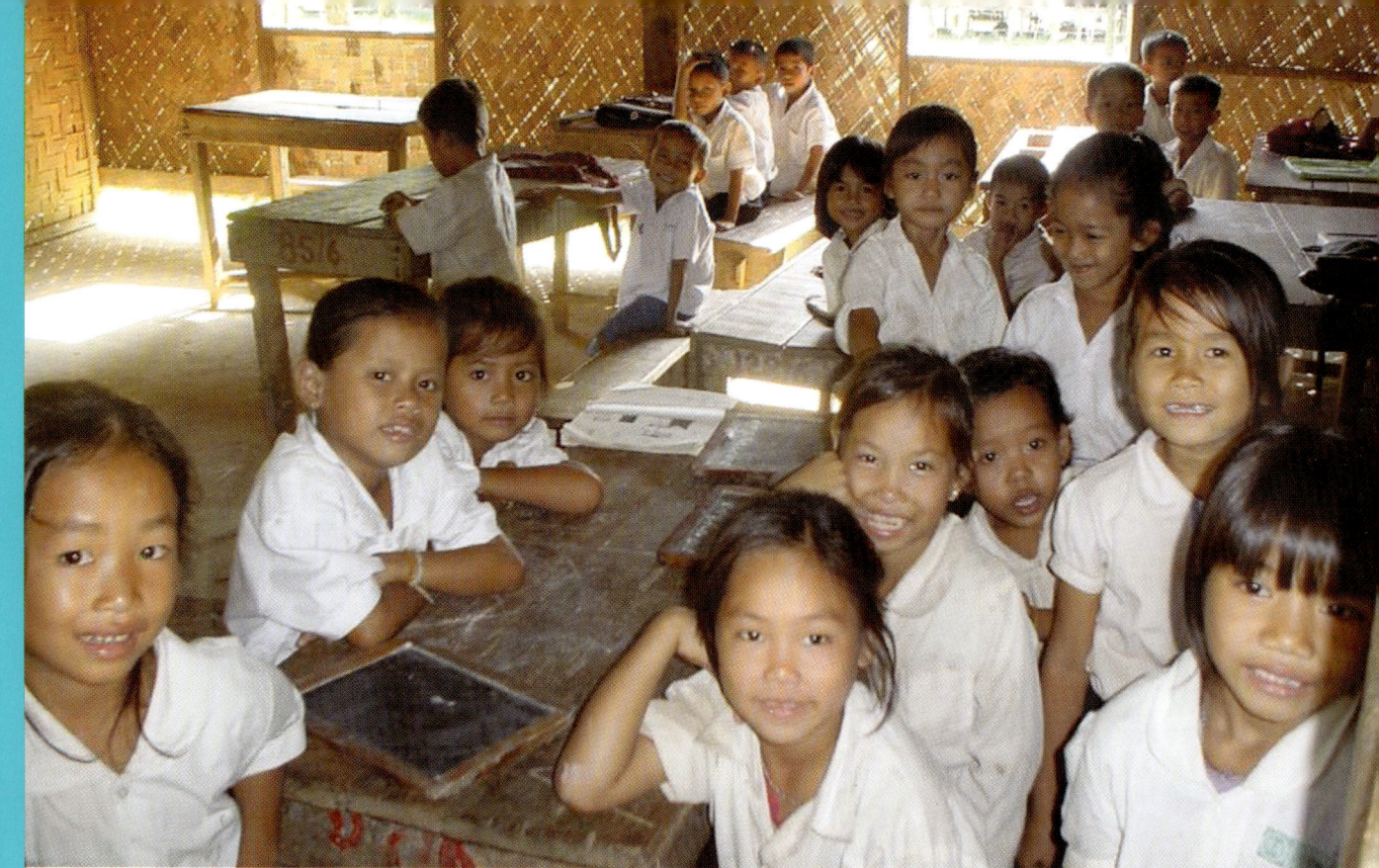

More than 75% of schoolchildren in the Lao People's Democratic Republic have been periodically dewormed

4. A solid foundation exists for programme implementation.

The past 10 years of work on NTDs in the region, particularly on LF elimination, has resulted in the establishment of a solid foundation for all NTD activities. Disease-specific interventions that are just starting can build on the planning, logistics, monitoring and evaluation capacity generated by the LF programme, though support is needed to further develop this capacity.

However, the crux of programming for many NTDs is mass drug administration, which involves distribution of medicines by community health-care workers and/or teachers. Therefore, the main interventions rely on an existing infrastructure that is accustomed to campaign-based programmes such as the Expanded Programme on Immunization and malaria bednet distribution.

5. Immediate results can be seen as NTDs are eliminated.

NTDs slated for elimination, such as leprosy, LF trachoma and yaws, need only a few more years of support to complete interventions to verify elimination. Within the next five years, positive results are expected as maps of endemic countries begin to shrink.

Investing in the region: building on existing success

NTD programming has a long and successful history in the Asia Pacific region that will play an important role in eliminating and controlling the diseases. Eight countries in the region have already drafted national integrated NTD plans with corresponding budgets, and 10 more are expected to formulate such plans in the near future. Nearly half of the necessary budget for NTD programmes comes from national governments, bilateral donors and the private sector. The Asia Pacific region has catalysed additional pharmaceutical donations by creating national plans and budget line items in many countries.

Past regional successes:

- Elimination of LF has been verified in China, the Republic of Korea and Solomon Islands.
- A total of 11 countries have reduced LF to elimination levels and are in the surveillance stage before verification.
- Leprosy has been eliminated (less than one case per 10 000 population) across the Asia Pacific region. Only three countries in the Western Pacific still need to eliminate it at national level.
- India eliminated yaws in 2006.
- Five countries – Cambodia, the Democratic Republic of Korea, the Lao People's Democratic Republic, Myanmar and Tuvalu – have achieved the global WHO target of at least 75% deworming coverage of school-age children.

For many countries in the Asia Pacific region, external funds will assist with the "last mile" of programming for diseases that can be eliminated. Much progress has already been made in the last 10 years. For a small number of countries, NTD programming will usher in an integrated plan to meet the global and regional guidelines for eliminating and controlling these diseases.

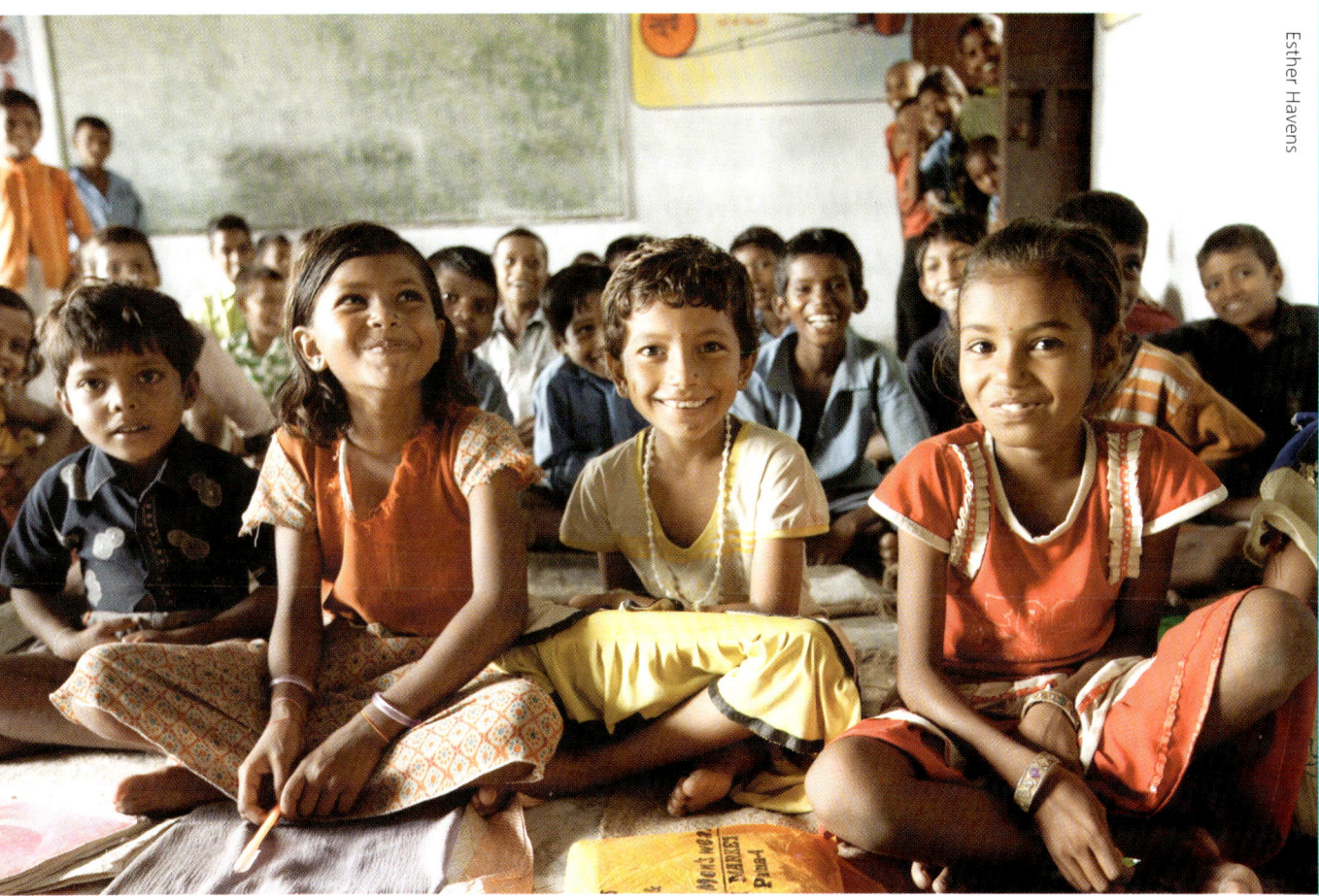

Children from Ghorahuan School in Bihar, India, actively participate in a deworming programme.

References

Addiss DG, Brady MA. Morbidity management in the global programme to eliminate lymphatic filariasis: a review of the scientific literature. Filaria Journal. 2007; 6, 2. doi:10.1186/1475-2883-6-2

Baird S, Hick JH, Kremer M, Miguel E. Worms at work: long-run impacts of child health gains. Berkeley: University of California at Berkeley; 2011

Bethony J, Brooker S, Albonico M, Geiger SM, Loukas A, Diemert D, et al.Soil-transmitted helminth infections: ascariasis, trichuriasis, and hookworm. Lancet. 2006; 367(9521), 1521–32. doi:10.1016/S0140–6736(06)68653–4

Brooker S, Hotez PJ, Bundy DAP. Hookworm-related anaemia among pregnant women: a systematic review. PLoS Negl Trop Dis. 2008; 2(9), e291. doi:10.1371/journal.pntd.0000291

Chu BK, Hooper PJ, Bradley MH, McFarland DA, Ottesen EA. The economic benefits resulting from the first 8 years of the Global Programme to Eliminate Lymphatic Filariasis (2000-2007). PLoS Negl Trop Dis. 2010; 4(6), e708. doi:10.1371/journal. pntd.0000708

Conteh L, Engels T, Molyneux DH. Socioeconomic aspects of neglected tropical diseases. Lancet. 2010; 375(9710), 239–47. doi:10.1016/S0140-6736(09)61422-7

Frick KD, Hanson CL, Jacobson GA. Global burden of trachoma and economics of the disease. Am J Trop Med Hyg. 2003; 69(5 Suppl), 1–10.

Goldman AS, Guisinger VH, Aikins M, Amarillo MLE, Belizario VY, Garshong B et al. National mass drug administration costs for lymphatic filariasis elimination. PLoS Negl Trop Dis. 2007;1(1), e67. doi:10.1371/journal.pntd.0000067

Larocque R, Casapia M, Gotuzzo E, Gyorkos TW. Relationship between intensity of soil-transmitted helminth infections and anemia during pregnancy. The Am J Trop Med Hyg. 2005; 73(4), 783–9.

Miguel E, Kremer M. Worms: identifying impacts on education and health in the presence of treatment externalities. Econometrica. 2004; 72(1), 159–217. doi:10.1111/j.1468-0262.2004.00481.x

Montresor A, Cong DT, Sinuon M, Tsuyuoka R, Chanthavisouk C, Strandgaard H et al. Large-scale preventive chemotherapy for the control of helminth infection in Western Pacific countries: six years later. PLoS Negl Trop Dis. 2008; 2(8), e278. doi:10.1371/journal.pntd.0000278

Ottesen EA, Hooper PJ, Bradley M, Biswas G. The global programme to eliminate lymphatic filariasis: health impact after 8 years. PLoS Negl Trop Dis. 2008; 2(10), e317. doi:10.1371/journal.pntd.0000317

Preventive chemotherapy in human helminthiasis. Geneva: World Health Organization; 2006 (http://whqlibdoc.who.int/publications/2006/9241547103_eng.pdf, accessed 29 November 2013).

Ramaiah KD, Das PK, Michael E, Guyatt H. The economic burden of lymphatic filariasis in India. Parasitology today. 2000; 16(6), 251–3

Weiss MG. Stigma and the social burden of neglected tropical diseases. PLoS Negl Trop Dis. 2008; 2(5), e237. doi:10.1371/journal.pntd.0000237

Appendix A
NTDs by country

Countries and Areas	Lymphatic filariasis Needs MDA	Schisto-somiasis Needs MDA	Trachoma Endemic	Yaws Endemic	Leprosy Above elimination threshold	Leishma-niasis Endemic	Soil-transmitted helminthiases Needs MDA	Foodborne trematodiases Endemic
South-East Asia Region								
Bangladesh	✓					✓	✓	
Bhutan						✓	✓	
India	✓		✓			✓	✓	✓
Indonesia	✓	✓		✓			✓	
The Democratic People's Republic of Korea							✓	
Maldives	✓							
Myanmar	✓		✓				✓	
Nepal	✓		✓			✓	✓	
Sri Lanka	✓							
Thailand	✓							✓
Timor-Leste	✓			✓			✓	
Western Pacific Region								
American Samoa	✓							
Australia			✓					
Brunei Darussalam	✓							
Cambodia	✓	✓	✓				✓	✓
China		✓	✓			✓	✓	✓

Countries and Areas	Lymphatic filariasis	Schisto-somiasis	Trachoma	Yaws	Leprosy	Leishma-niasis	Soil-transmitted helminthiases	Foodborne trematodiases
	Needs MDA	Needs MDA	Endemic	Endemic	Above elimination threshold	Endemic	Needs MDA	Endemic
Cook Islands	✓							
The Federated States of Micronesia	✓				✓		✓	
Fiji	✓		✓				✓	
French Polynesia	✓							
Guam								
Hong Kong (China)								
Japan								
Kiribati	✓		✓		✓		✓	
The Republic of Korea								✓
The Lao People's Democratic Republic	✓	✓	✓				✓	✓
Macao (China)								
Malaysia	✓						✓	
The Marshall Islands	✓				✓		✓	
Mongolia								
Nauru			✓				✓	
New Caledonia	✓							
New Zealand								
Niue	✓							
The Commonwealth of the Northern Mariana Islands								
Palau	✓							
Papua New Guinea	✓		✓	✓			✓	✓
The Philippines	✓	✓					✓	✓
The Pitcairn Islands								
Samoa	✓						✓	
Singapore								
Solomon Islands			✓	✓			✓	
Tokelau								
Tonga	✓						✓	
Tuvalu	✓						✓	
Vanuatu	✓		✓	✓			✓	
Viet Nam	✓		✓				✓	✓
Wallis and Futuna	✓							
TOTAL	31	5	14	5	3	5	25	9

MDA = mass drug administration.
Source: World Health Organization.

Appendix B
Disease Profiles

Foodborne trematodiases (FBT)

What are FBT?
- FBT are parasitic infections caused by liver and lung flukes that are transmitted through eating raw or undercooked freshwater fish, crab or aquatic vegetables that contain larvae.
- Infections can cause severe clinical manifestations, including chronic liver disease, cancer and lung disease.

Where is it found in the Asia Pacific region?
- At least nine countries are endemic for at least one FBT – Cambodia, China, India, the Lao People's Democratic Republic, Papua New Guinea, the Philippines, the Republic of Korea, Thailand and Viet Nam.

Who is at risk?
- At least 1 million people are at risk for at least one FBT.

What can be done?
- Mass drug administration is recommended in high-burden areas.
- In low-burden areas, individual case detection and treatment needs to be provided through the primary health care system.
- Health education is necessary for sustainable control, as people need to be persuaded to change their eating habits.
- Collaboration with the agricultural sector is necessary to improve practices of deworming infected animals and managing livestock and fisheries.

What is the status in the Asia Pacific region?
- Mapping of FBT is complete in four countries – China, the Lao People's Democratic Republic, the Republic of Korea and Viet Nam.
- Mass drug administration or selective treatment is continuing in Cambodia, China, India, the Lao People's Democratic Republic, the Philippines, the Republic of Korea, Thailand and Viet Nam.

Leishmaniasis

What is leishmaniasis?
- Visceral leishmaniasis, also known as kala azar, is a disease caused by parasites transmitted through the bites of sandflies.
- It attacks the internal organs and is usually fatal within two years if left untreated.

Where is it found in the Asia Pacific region?
- It is endemic in five countries: Bangladesh, Bhutan, China, India and Nepal.

What can be done?
- The goal is to eliminate the disease (less than one new case per 10 000 population at risk) by 2015 in Bangladesh, India and Nepal.
- Disease can be reduced through active case detection and early treatment.
- Controlling vectors and reservoirs of hosts are also necessary as part of a comprehensive approach to disease control.

What is the status in the Asia Pacific region?
- Bangladesh, India and Nepal are implementing early case finding, delivering oral treatment and implementing vector control measures.
- China is implementing screening and treatment of infected persons, especially after outbreaks.

Leprosy

What is leprosy?
- Leprosy is a bacterial infection that slowly progresses to affect skin, peripheral nerves, the upper respiratory tract, eyes and other organs. Most people have a natural immunity to the disease, but those who are left untreated can develop permanent disabilities and often are subjected to discrimination and exclusion from society.

Where is it found in the Asia Pacific region?
- Three countries have not yet eliminated leprosy as a public health problem – Kiribati, the Marshall Islands and the Federated States of Micronesia.
- Other countries in the region, such as China, India and the Philippines, still need to address high numbers of cases.

Who is at risk?
- There were 129 091 people with leprosy in the Asia Pacific region (2010), with 9.39 new cases per 100 000 people detected in South-East Asia and 0.29 new cases per 100 000 people in the Western Pacific in 2009.

What can be done?
- The regional goal is to eliminate leprosy as a public health problem in all countries and areas by 2016.
- Patients need to be able to access early diagnosis through primary health care services, where they can receive free multidrug therapy.

What is the status in the Asia Pacific region?
- Elimination as a public health problem was achieved in 1991 (less than one case per 10 000 population) at a regional level.
- Countries and areas that have achieved elimination targets now aim to decrease the number of cases with disability through early detection and treatment.

Lymphatic filariasis (LF)

What is LF?
- LF is a crippling, mosquito-borne infection that can result in swollen limbs and breasts, genital damage and thickened, hardened skin.

Where is it found in the Asia Pacific region?
- It is endemic in 31 countries and areas.

Who is at risk?
- About 927 million people require mass drug administration to eliminate LF.

What can be done?
- LF is slated to be eliminated globally by 2020.
- In communities at risk, medicines are administered yearly for at least five years to break the cycle of transmission.
- People with lymphoedema need access to chronic care through the primary health care system, and people with hydrocele need access to surgery.

What is the status in the Asia Pacific region?
- China, the Republic of Korea and Solomon Islands have eliminated LF.
- Eleven other countries have eliminated LF and are pending verification.
- A total of 17 countries have continuing mass drug administration.
- Three countries still need to determine if they are endemic.
- Papua New Guinea and Timor-Leste need to pay more attention to LF, with success dependent upon the ability of national LF programmes to synergize with other programmes and engage a multipartner coalition.

Schistosomiasis

What is schistosomiasis?
- Schistosomiasis is a parasitic disease caused by trematode flatworms and is transmitted by eggs excreted in human faeces or urine, which contaminate water sources in areas that lack adequate sanitation. Humans are infected through the penetration of the skin by infective larvae carried by contaminated water.
- It can cause anaemia, stunting and developmental problems in children, with long-term complications, including severe liver pathology.

Where is it found in the Asia Pacific region?
- It is endemic in five countries — Cambodia, China, the Lao People's Democratic Republic, Indonesia and the Philippines.

Who is at risk?
- About 4.2 million people are at risk, with 620 000 school-age children requiring deworming.

What can be done?
- In areas of high risk of infection, at least 75% of school-age children should be given deworming drugs to quickly reduce morbidity.
- In order to sustain reductions in morbidity, health education and water and sanitation improvements must also be performed. These steps require collaboration with other programmes such as education, environment and poverty reduction.
- Snail control and improvements in agriculture to distance humans from animal hosts are often necessary to interrupt transmission.

What is the status in the Asia Pacific region?
- All five endemic countries are conducting mass deworming.
- Mass deworming needs to be sustained until water, sanitation and farming practices improve.

Soil-transmitted helminthiases (STH)

What are STH?
- STH, commonly known as intestinal worms, infect the intestines, leading to anaemia, vitamin A deficiencies, stunting, malnutrition, impaired development and intestinal obstruction.
- People are infected through ingesting eggs from contaminated soil or by larvae penetrating the skin.

Where is it found in the Asia Pacific region?
- At least 25 countries and areas need mass drug distribution to control STH.
- Infections are widely distributed and linked to a lack of clean water, proper sanitation and poverty in general.

Who is at risk?
- At least 471 million children require deworming.
- School-age children are most at risk from morbidity since they usually have the highest burden of worms in a community.
- Preschool-age children also are at high risk since they have high loads of worms.
- Women of childbearing age are considered a high-risk group since they are at risk of suffering from anaemia, which can result in low birthweight infants.

What can be done?
- In areas of high risk of infection, at least 75% of preschool-age and school-age children should be given deworming drugs once or twice a year to reduce morbidity. quickly
- Mass deworming can be integrated with other health programmes, such as the Expanded Programme on Immunization which targets small children and mothers.
- In order to sustain reductions in morbidity, and finally interrupt transmission, health education and water and sanitation improvements must also be performed. These steps require collaboration with other sectors such as education and environment.

What is the status in the Asia Pacific region?
- Five countries have achieved the global target of >75% deworming coverage of school-age children and need to maintain it until water and sanitation improvements occur.
- Thirteen more countries have reported deworming of school-aged children but need to scale up to provide full coverage.
- At least seven countries have not yet reported mass deworming of school-age children.
- Two countries reported high deworming coverage in preschool-age children.
- Two countries reported deworming in women of childbearing age, but all countries need to scale up access to this target group.

Trachoma

What is trachoma?
- Trachoma is an infection of the eye that is spread from person to person by direct contact. It results in the scarring of the upper eyelid, which leads to blindness.

Where is it found in the Asia Pacific region?
- It is endemic in at least 14 countries.

Who is at risk?
- At least 100 million people are at risk.

What can be done?
- The goal is to eliminate blinding trachoma by 2020 globally, including provision of surgery to everyone with trichiasis.[10]
- Mass administration of antibiotics is recommended in communities with high prevalence. Hygiene and environmental improvements are also necessary as part of a comprehensive approach to interrupt transmission.

What is the status in the Asia Pacific region?
- Cambodia, China, India, Myanmar, Nepal and Viet Nam aim to achieve elimination by 2016.
- Mass antibiotic distribution is continuing in Australia, Cambodia, India, the Lao People's Democratic Republic, Myanmar and Nepal.
- Surveys are needed to better understand the distribution of the infection in Fiji, Kiribati, Nauru, Papua New Guinea, Solomon Islands and Vanuatu.

---

[10] Trichiasis is caused by abnormally positioned eyelashes that grow toward the eye, touching the cornea, potentially leading to opacification and blindness

Yaws

What is yaws?
- Yaws is a bacterial infection that is transmitted from person to person through highly contagious skins lesions. It can lead to disfigurements and disability of the skin and bones.

Where is it found in the Asia Pacific region?
- Based on historical evidence, five countries are endemic – Indonesia, Papua New Guinea, Solomon Islands, Timor-Leste and Vanuatu.
- Since yaws thrives in warm, moist tropical climates, there might be other Pacific island countries that also have experienced cases of yaws.

Who is at risk?
- An unknown number of people are at risk, mostly those who live in conditions of poverty, where overcrowding and poor hygiene help spread the disease.

What can be done?
- The regional target is yaws elimination by 2020.
- Yaws can be treated by a single injection of long-lasting benzathine benzyl penicillin. The strategy is to find cases early and to treat the patients and their close contacts, such as family and neighbours. Surveillance is then needed to ensure infections do not re-emerge.
- A new strategy is to use azithromycin as part of mass community medicine distribution in highly endemic areas.

What is the status in the Asia Pacific region?
- India was endemic for yaws, but it was eliminated in 2006.
- Indonesia and Timor-Leste have continuing case finding and treatment.
- Vanuatu and Solomon Islands will formulate national action plans in 2012 while Papua New Guinea needs to be mapped.

Other NTDs

Other NTDs also exist in the Asia Pacific region. Countries and areas need technical assistance to support better assessments of disease distribution and burden as well as to formulate and implement control strategies.
- **Echinococcosis,** a tapeworm infection that causes cysts in the liver and lungs in humans, is endemic in China and Mongolia. The tapeworm lives in sheep and dogs and accidentally infects humans when they ingest eggs through contact with sheep and dogs or consume vegetables and water contaminated with dog faeces.
- **Taeniasis/cysticercosis** is a tapeworm infection that is transmitted to humans through the consumption of undercooked pork. It causes cysts in the central nervous system, which can cause epilepsy. It is a public health problem in China, Mongolia and Viet Nam.
- **Buruli ulcer** is a chronic necrotizing skin disease caused by a bacterium similar to that which causes tuberculosis and leprosy. Infection leads to large ulcers, usually on the legs or arms and, if treatment is delayed, long-term disabilities. At least five countries in the region have a history of Buruli ulcer cases, but more information is needed to truly know the extent of the distribution.

Appendix C
Specific resource requirements

Table 1 Budget gaps for South-East Asia and Western Pacific Region NTD initiatives, by region

	Estimated total 5-year budget (US$)	Funding gap (US$)	Funding gap (% of total)	Funding committed (% of total)
South-East Asia Region subtotal	153 000 000	76 000 000	50%	50%
Western Pacific Region subtotal	89 913 611	44 977 794	50%	50%
Asia Pacific Region Total	242 913 611	120 977 794	50%	50%

Above figures do not include budgets for Brunei Darussalam, China, India, Japan, Malaysia, New Caledonia and the Republic of Korea or regional costs for the Western Pacific Regional Office and the South-East Asia Regional Office.
Source: World Health Organization.

Table 2 Budget gaps for the Western Pacific Region NTD Initiative, by objective and year

Year	Objective 1: Advocacy (US$)	Objective 2: Programme Management (US$)	Objective 3: Access (US$)	Objective 4: Monitoring and Evaluation (US$)	Objective 5: Research (US$)	Regional Costs (US$)	TOTAL
2012	92 704	898 744	5 466 414	1 242 388	250 000	1 544 372	9 494 622
2013	77 704	879 804	8 373 184	966 555	250 000	1 927 509	12 474 756
2014	77 704	947 491	7 915 684	721 268	250 000	2 077 260	11 989 407
2015	77 704	856 731	7 744 052	1 374 057	250 000	2 241 986	12 544 530
2016	72 304	336 531	5 543 002	383 769	50 000	2 423 185	8 808 791
TOTAL	398 120	3 919 301	35 042 336	4 688 037	1 050 000	10 214 312	55 312 106

Source: World Health Organization.

Table 3 Budget gaps for the Western Pacific Region NTD Initiative, by objective and disease

Disease	Objective 1: Advocacy (US$)	Objective 2: Programme Management (US$)	Objective 3: Access (US$)	Objective 4: Monitoring and Evaluation (US$)	Objective 5: Research (US$)	Regional (US$)	TOTAL
LF	151 475	733 310	4 559 210	1 504 638	140 000	2 697 475	9 786 108
STH	64 355	2 245 400	18 578 203	1 308 018	20 000	1 348 737	23 564 713
Schistosomiasis	23 290	63 585	4 192 824	82 343	30 000	1 348 737	5 740 779
Trachoma	0	7 819	1 310 204	534 707	20 000	0	1 872 730
FBT	39 000	434 187	4 684 895	848 333	840 000	674 369	7 520 784
Yaws	0	0	430 000	25 000	0	674 369	1 129 369
Leprosy	120 000	435 000	1 287 000	384 998	0	3 470 625	5 697 623
TOTAL	398 120	3 919 301	35 042 336	4 688 037	1 050 000	10 214 312	55 312 106

Source: World Health Organization.